Processed Food Addiction Cure

A Beginner's 3-Week Step-by-Step Guide with Sample Curated Recipes

mf

Disclaimer

By reading this disclaimer, you are accepting the terms of the disclaimer in full. If you disagree with this disclaimer, please do not read the guide.

All of the content within this guide is provided for informational and educational purposes only, and should not be accepted as independent medical or other professional advice. The author is not a doctor, physician, nurse, mental health provider, or registered nutritionist/dietician. Therefore, using and reading this guide does not establish any form of a physician-patient relationship.

Always consult with a physician or another qualified health provider with any issues or questions you might have regarding any sort of medical condition. Do not ever disregard any qualified professional medical advice or delay seeking that advice because of anything you have read in this guide. The information in this guide is not intended to be any sort of medical advice and should not be used in lieu of any medical advice by a licensed and qualified medical professional.

The information in this guide has been compiled from a variety of known sources. However, the author cannot attest to or guarantee the accuracy of each source and thus should not be held liable for any errors or omissions.

You acknowledge that the publisher of this guide will not be held liable for any loss or damage of any kind incurred as a result of this guide or the reliance on any information provided within this guide. You acknowledge and agree that you assume all risk and responsibility for any action you undertake in response to the information in this guide.

Using this guide does not guarantee any particular result (e.g., weight loss or a cure). By reading this guide, you acknowledge that there are no guarantees to any specific outcome or results you can expect.

All product names, diet plans, or names used in this guide are for identification purposes only and are the property of their respective owners. The use of these names does not imply endorsement. All other trademarks cited herein are the property of their respective owners.

Where applicable, this guide is not intended to be a substitute for the original work of this diet plan and is, at most, a supplement to the original work for this diet plan and never a direct substitute. This guide is a personal expression of the facts of that diet plan.

Where applicable, persons shown in the cover images are stock photography models and the publisher has obtained the rights to use the images through license agreements with third-party stock image companies.

Table of Contents

Introduction

Processed food addiction is a serious problem in the United States. It's estimated that up to 70% of all processed foods are addictive, and this number is only going to continue increasing as food manufacturers become more creative with their products.

What does processed food addiction mean? Similar to any form of addiction, being addicted to processed foods means experiencing difficulties in curbing the desire to consume them, which even our brains can't say no to. Processed foods are as addictive to humans as drugs and alcohol.

This particular addiction has serious health consequences including obesity, diabetes, heart disease, hypertension, and cancer, to name some. It also affects the quality of life in other areas such as moods or emotional well-being, as well as social relationships.

The bottom line is that processed foods can lead to critical health problems for millions of people around the world if they aren't properly educated about what's happening inside their bodies when consuming these products. That's why it's crucial to know how processed foods work on a biological level.

In this guide, you will learn how processed foods work on a biological level, what to look for in the food items themselves, and provide three actionable steps that can help you beat processed food addiction.

In this quick start guide, you will discover...

- What processed food is all about
- What processed food addiction is
- Why it's hard to give up consuming processed foods
- How processed foods consumption affect the brain and the body
- A 3-week plan to help you beat processed food addiction

All About Processed Food

Processed food is any type of food that has been modified from its natural state. This includes foods that have been processed by humans, such as cooking, canning, freezing, or milling, or foods that have been processed by machines, such as extrusion and injection molding.

The most common processed foods are:

- Baked goods: bread and pastries
- Canned foods: fruits, vegetables, soups, and meats
- Convenience foods: frozen dinners or takeout
- Dairy products: cheese and yogurt
- Drinks: soda and juice
- Fast food

There are also things known as "Food Additives." These are substances added to food to improve its taste, color, texture, or shelf life. These additives can be natural or artificial.

Some common food additives include:

- Artificial flavors and colors
- Preservatives, such as BHA and BHT

- Emulsifiers, such as soy lecithin
- Stabilizers, such as carrageenan
- Sweeteners, such as high-fructose corn syrup

One easy method to determine if something is processed is to look at the ingredient list on the label. If you see a long list of ingredients that you don't recognize, then it's likely processed.

Another simpler method is by asking yourself, "Would I be able to make this food myself at home?" If the answer is no, then it's likely processed.

About ultra-processed foods

The majority of processed foods in the U.S. are ultra-processed foods. These are foods that contain industrial ingredients and have been heavily processed to the point where they no longer resemble their original form. It is estimated in 2016 that ultra-processed foods make up 78% of the American diet.

One example is soft drinks, which contain natural flavors, high fructose corn syrup, caramel color, citric acid, phosphoric acid, caffeine powder, etc. Just look at those ingredients and ask yourself if you could make that drink at home. The answer is most likely no.

Another example would be a candy bar, which consists of some kind of chocolate coating with sugar or cocoa solids on top. The rest of it includes milk powders and other types of sugars including maltitol sweetener along with polydextrose as well as artificial flavorings such as vanillin. Again, this is something that you would be hard-pressed to make at home. It also includes emulsifiers like lecithin and artificial colors like FD&C Red 40.

Ultra-processed foods are linked to a number of health problems, including obesity, diabetes, heart disease, hypertension, and cancer. They're also incredibly addictive, and it can be very hard to quit eating them when you know they're bad for you.

Why are processed foods so unhealthy?

Processed foods are unhealthy for the following reasons. To put it simply, they are high in sugar, unhealthy fats, and salt.

Sugar is unhealthy because it is devoid of nutrients. It doesn't provide any vitamins or minerals that the body needs to thrive and fight off diseases, leaving the body starved for what it actually needs in order to function properly.

It can also cause many health problems such as obesity, heart disease, diabetes, and cancer because when sugar is consumed constantly, the body becomes insulin resistant, making it difficult to process it.

This means that all of the sugar stays in our system, causing us to gain weight and become unhealthy. Another reason that sugar is so bad for us is that it messes with our hormones.

When we eat too much sugar, it causes our blood sugar levels to increase, making us feel good by giving our body a rush of endorphins.

However, when we consume sugary food constantly throughout the day, our blood sugar levels will spike and then crash back down to low levels. This can cause more sugary food cravings in order to raise the blood sugar back up again. This creates a vicious cycle that can be hard to break.

Unhealthy fats, most commonly known as trans fats, contribute to the risk of diabetes and heart diseases by increasing bad cholesterol levels. Other health problems such as cancer and obesity can also be linked back to trans-fats.

Salt is unhealthy because it causes us to retain water and raises our blood pressure. When we have high blood pressure, it puts stress on our hearts and increases our risk of heart disease and stroke. Too much salt can also cause kidney stones and stomach cancer.

Moreover, processed foods are full of artificial chemicals. These chemicals can be harmful to your body, and over time they can contribute to health problems. For example, artificial colors are linked to cancer, while preservatives can cause organ damage. A study by the University of Liverpool, published in the journal Food Research International, found that some artificial colors can even cause hyperactivity and other behavioral problems.

You should always read food labels before buying something packaged to make sure you don't buy foods with added chemicals! For example, if it says "sodium benzoate" on a label, you should put it back on the shelf.

As a reminder, if your grandma wouldn't recognize an ingredient as being something edible that she knows and loves then you probably shouldn't be eating it!

Lastly, beyond just being unhealthy for your physical body, processed foods are extremely addictive, which is something you might be struggling with. Processed foods are also addictive because they contain refined sugars, which trigger the release of dopamine in our brains. Dopamine is a neurotransmitter that makes you feel good and can lead to cravings for more processed food.

Processed Food Addiction and How It Affects Your Brain

Our society has become more vigilant when it comes to protecting the youth from drug addiction. However, we don't realize that there is another form of addiction that we become negligent of, that is an addiction to food, particularly processed food. This type of addiction not only affects adults but also children, even toddlers. There is various research and studies that support this, one of which proves how this food addiction usually spans from early development in the uterus until adulthood.

How the Brain Is Triggered

Processed food, in general, contains ingredients such as fat, salt, and sugar—all of which are not only known to make processed food taste better but also to trigger the release of natural opiates. Salt, in particular, has been found to function similarly to how addictive drugs do. One study even referred to it as the salt appetite.

These staple ingredients in processed food not only make them taste better but also trigger the brain to produce natural opiates called endogenous opioids. There are two ways these opioids help the body—to bind either to a so-called pain pathway or a reward pathway. When the opioids bind to the reward pathway, it results in the production of dopamine. When they bind to the pain pathway, the brain produces endorphins.

Dopamine and Endorphins

Dopamine and endorphins, as we all know, are brain chemicals that provide support to the body. Dopamine provides the feeling of being rewarded, while endorphins provide the feeling to cope with pain and stress.

When dopamine is released, the body instantly feels pleasure, sort of feeling high. The euphoric feeling is sustained when you keep providing your body with the reward-binding opiates, which is processed food. Once you're finished eating, the production of dopamine also stops. Naturally, the brain will want to repeat this process because of its effects, thus the impulse to once again provide the source that triggered the opiates. This is how addiction to processed food and even drugs happens.

In one example, the Flamin' Hot Cheetos which has the red pepper spice flavor triggers the receptors in the body that respond to spice and heat. This results in the release of natural opioids to balance the heat, binding to the pain pathway, resulting in the release of endorphins to help you feel better after consuming something that "burned" your stomach. It's a feel-good feeling, along with the flavors—spicy and salty.

Aside from that, there is also evidence that suggests that processed food, or in particular, those from fast food restaurants have these specific components that make them addictive, not much different from how cocaine and heroin work.

Eventually, this develops into a habit of eating just to achieve the same feeling repetitively. Aside from that, most processed food also falls under the term "hyper-palatable," coined by former FDA commissioner Dr. David Kessler. They are called such because, again, of the pleasurable feeling they trigger when consumed, it becomes a habit to consume them, which may eventually lead to addiction.

A Brief Introduction to Healthy Foods

Now that you have learned about processed foods, you may now be wondering what you should eat instead. The good news is that there are plenty of healthy and delicious foods out there that you can eat instead!

Some of our favorites include fruits, vegetables, whole grains, lean proteins, and healthy fats. These foods are all packed with nutrients your body needs to stay healthy and they don't contain any unhealthy ingredients like sugar, unhealthy fats, or salt. What do all these foods have in common? They only consist of one or two ingredients and they are all unprocessed!

Fruits

Fruits are a great source of vitamins, minerals, and antioxidants, which can help protect your body from disease. They also contain natural sugars, which are a healthier type of sugar than the refined sugars found in processed foods. Some of our favorites include berries, apples, and bananas.

Eating a variety of fruits is important for getting the right mix of nutrients. Be sure to include some that are high in fiber, like berries and pears, as well as those that are low in sugar, like cucumbers and tomatoes.

Here is a list of some other healthy fruits to include in your diet:

- Kiwi
- Papaya
- Pineapple
- Mango
- Apricot
- Cantaloupe
- Watermelon

Vegetables

Vegetables are an important part of a healthy diet and they are packed with nutrients like vitamins, minerals, and antioxidants. They also contain no unhealthy ingredients like sugar, unhealthy fats, or salt.

Vegetables are packed with nutrients, fiber, vitamins, and minerals that are essential for good health. They also contain antioxidants, which can help protect your body from disease. Some of our favorites include dark leafy greens, carrots, and tomatoes.

Here is a list of some other vegetables that you should include in your diet.

- Bell peppers
- Broccoli
- Cabbage
- Cauliflower
- Green beans
- Kale
- Lettuce
- Mushrooms
- Onions
- Peas
- Spinach
- Squash (summer & winter)
- Sweet potatoes
- Tomatoes

Whole Grains

Whole grains are a great source of fiber, vitamins, and minerals. Fiber is important for digestion and helps keep us feeling full after eating. Whole grains also contain antioxidants that can help protect our bodies from disease. Some of our favorites include oats, quinoa, and brown rice.

Here is a list of some other whole grains that you should include in your diet:

- Barley

- Buckwheat (Kasha)
- Bulgur
- Millet
- Wild rice
- Oats
- Quinoa
- Rice, brown or white
- Rye
- Sorghum
- Teff

The US Department of Agriculture (USDA) is also a good source for a comprehensive list of whole grains. The list is included in the programs for child nutrition, but it could also be used as a guide for adults.

The USDA website provides information on the nutrient content and health benefits of many different types of whole grains. It is important to remember that not all whole grains provide equal nutrients; some have more nutrients than others. Be sure to do your research before making any changes to your diet.

Lean Proteins

Proteins are essential for building muscle mass and repairing tissue. They are also a good source of energy. Lean proteins come from animal sources or plant-based sources like legumes or nuts. Our favorites include grilled chicken, salmon, and spinach.

Here is a list of some other lean proteins that you can include in your diet:

- Beef, flank steak
- Pork, loin or tenderloin
- Turkey, breast, or thigh
- Chicken, all parts
- Eggs
- Tuna, fresh or canned in water
- Salmon, fresh or frozen
- Shrimp, fresh or frozen
- Lentils and beans (black, kidney, garbanzo)
- Nuts (almonds, peanuts, walnuts)
- Seeds (pumpkin, sunflower)

Healthy Fats

There are three types of healthy fats: unsaturated, saturated, and trans fat.

Unsaturated fats come from plant sources like olive oil or avocado and can help lower bad cholesterol levels in our bodies while also providing essential vitamins and minerals to us that we need for good health.

Saturated fats come mainly from animal products but some plant-based foods contain them as well, such as coconut oil, palm kernel oil, and cocoa butter. These kinds of unhealthy fats should be eaten sparingly due to their link with increased risk for heart disease when consumed regularly.

Trans fat is a manmade type of fat found mostly in processed food items like crackers, chips, or baked goods made with partially hydrogenated oils or margarine. Trans fats are the unhealthiest type of fat and should be avoided at all costs!

Here is a list of some healthy fats that you can include in your diet:
- Olive oil
- Coconut oil
- Avocado
- Nuts (almonds, peanuts, walnuts)
- Seeds (flax, chia, hemp)
- Butter, ghee, or clarified butter
- Margarine, trans-fat free
- Fish oils
- Dairy (yogurt, cheese)

Week 1 – Retrain the Brain

One of the best ways to curb processed food addiction is by changing the way you think about food. You need to start viewing food as something that fuels your body and helps you stay healthy, not something to mainly make you feel happy or rewarded.

Remember what food is for

Food is about providing nutrition, and keeping the body healthy and nourished. Without food, the body will not be able to function properly. However, you also need to remember to pick the right food. Just because something tastes good and fills you up doesn't mean it's healthy.

Processed food contains ingredients that are meant to make you want to eat it habitually, without much regard for your health. Thus, it's important to stay disciplined in controlling your urges to eat processed food.

Consider your health

Every time you are tempted to eat junk or processed food, remind yourself that they don't do you good. Consumption of processed food contributes to obesity, diabetes, and other diseases that hurt your health. These health conditions usually affect you for a long time.

Treating these conditions linked to processed food addiction may also be very financially draining. Some may require you to be on maintenance medication. Some may require more intrusive or painful remedies.

Think about who you are letting down by not eating healthy, and how this attitude will affect your health for a long time.

Involve your family

Curbing processed food addiction may be best done by finding someone who can both hold you accountable for your goals and who can support you in achieving them. It may be hard to involve your entire family in the program, but informing them of your choices and your preference will help you stay motivated.

For example, do your groceries separately from the rest of the family. That way, you won't have to be tempted by seeing the bag of chips lined up on the shelves in the grocery store. At home, ask your family to store these processed foods away from your usual storage, so that you won't have to worry about seeing them and getting tempted to open one or have a bite.

Keep a food journal

One way to keep on track with your goal of retraining your brain is by keeping a food journal. List down your goals, recipes, and sample meal plans, as well as any other plans you have to help you keep motivated.

Once you have successfully started retraining your brain and seeing processed foods in a new light, you can move on to Week Two.

Week 2 – Choose Right

Now that week 1 is done, it's time to work on making the right choices.

Start getting rid of junk food

To keep you motivated, start getting rid of the junk and processed food in your pantry. You may either do it gradually or in one go, whatever works best for you. Review the food and ingredients lists in the previous chapter to give you a refresher on processed food, particularly frozen and canned goods.

The problem with addiction is the intense desire to keep doing what you're supposed to be avoiding. When you are finally out of processed food in your pantry, make sure that you don't replenish them, or find a way to make them inaccessible, especially if you don't live alone.

Stock up on good food items

Now that your pantry is clear of processed food, it's time to replenish it with better options: healthy food choices, such as fresh produce, fresh meat, and whole grains. Try also to avoid food with ingredients that are considered unhealthy, if you can. Also, choosing to go organic and natural is a great step to achieving your goal.

Make eating healthy exciting

Just because you choose to eat healthy doesn't mean food will not be fun to eat. Healthy food doesn't have to be boring or tasteless. There are a lot of fun recipes that you can try to spice up your appetite for healthy food.

Cooking your own meal will also make it more fun, as you can appreciate the food preparation process that goes through, and are able to understand how different it is when you're preparing fresh food versus processed food.

Don't be intimidated if you haven't tried preparing food following recipes that may seem sophisticated. Remember, all those ingredients are just food, nothing to worry about.

To motivate you, here are some basic tips when cooking for the first time:

- Start by washing your fruits and vegetables. This is important to remove any pesticides or chemicals that might be on the surface.
- Cut your vegetables into bite-sized pieces so they are easier to eat.

- Cook your proteins and grains in a healthy way. This might include grilling, baking, poaching, or boiling.
- Use healthy cooking oils such as avocado oil, coconut oil, or avocado oil when cooking. These oils are high in monounsaturated fats which are good for our health.
- Use herbs and spices to flavor your food instead of salt or sugar. This is a much healthier way to add flavor to your food.

Week 3 – Maintain Good Eating Habits

During the last week of this plan, focus on keeping good habits and avoiding bad ones, mainly food triggers. This refers to situations that may tempt you to break from your goal of eating clean. Remember, these situations don't always have to be negative, but they may still trigger your processed food addiction.

Examples include:

- stress
- boredom
- parties or gatherings

The list of triggers goes on and on. The important thing to remember is that they are all things you can avoid by planning ahead or creating new habits. Triggers cause us to act impulsively, which means we don't think about what it is that we're doing before making a decision. By avoiding these triggers completely or by having a plan in place, we can circumvent this and make healthier choices.

In addition to avoiding triggers, it's important to maintain the good habits that we've created over the past two weeks. This means cooking at home as often as possible, packing healthy snacks for when we're on the go, and staying active.

If you still have any hidden processed foods in your house, now is the time to get rid of them. Throw them away or give them to a friend who might be able to use them. The goal is to make our home environment as healthy as possible so that we are less likely to fall back into unhealthy eating habits.

The final step is to reward yourself for a job well done! Take the time every week or month to write down all of your successes and celebrate them. After you've completed this three-week plan, feel free to continue along with the healthy changes that have become a habit now.

Sample Recipes

This chapter contains healthy recipes. They are all simple and tasty, so give them a try!

Tuna Salad

Ingredients:

- 1/2 cup pecans
- 1 cup chicken breast, steamed and cubed
- 1 cup tuna in oil
- salt, to taste
- pepper, to taste

Instructions:

1. Mix all ingredients in a large bowl.
2. Add a dash of salt and pepper to taste.
3. Chill for at least an hour before serving.

Turkey with Avocado Salad

Ingredients:

- 1 lb. lean ground turkey
- 1 avocado, sliced
- 1 can black olives
- 2 heads romaine lettuce, hand rip to bite-sized pieces
- 2 tbsp. extra-virgin olive oil
- 1 tsp. balsamic vinegar
- 1/2 tsp. sea salt

Instructions:

1. Season turkey patties with salt. Place on and cook for 5 minutes on each side.
2. Set aside to cool before carving into bite-size pieces.
3. Place olives, lettuce, vinegar, and oil in a salad bowl. Toss all the ingredients together.
4. Garnish with avocado slices and burger pieces on top.
5. Serve and enjoy.

Grilled Tuna

Ingredients:

- tuna
- 4 tbsp. lemon juice
- 2 cloves garlic, minced
- salt
- pepper

Instructions:

1. Marinate tuna with garlic and lemon juice.
2. Season with salt and pepper.
3. Grill for 8-10 minutes.
4. Add more fresh ground pepper upon serving.
5. Serve and enjoy while hot.

Spinach Quiche

Ingredients:

- 1 lb. breakfast sausage
- 1/2 onion, diced
- 2 cups mushrooms, sliced
- 6 cups spinach, roughly chopped
- 12 eggs
- 1/4 to 1/2 cup full-fat coconut milk
- 1 tsp. garlic powder
- 1 tsp. Italian seasoning
- 1 tsp. salt
- 1 tsp. pepper

Instructions:

1. Preheat the oven to 400°F.
2. Heat a cast-iron pan or another oven-safe pan over medium heat.
3. Cook sausage and onion. Stir occasionally until sausage turns brown, about 7-8 minutes.
4. Add in mushrooms. Allow them to cook with the sausage until soft, for about 2 minutes. Remove from heat.
5. Crack eggs into a large bowl.
6. Add coconut milk. For a lighter and fluffier texture, use ½ cup. Use less for less coconut taste.
7. Whisk together well to get a light egg mixture.

8. Add spinach and seasonings to the bowl with the eggs.

9. Add the sausage mixture to the bowl with the rest of the ingredients.

10. Mix until everything is well blended.

11. Line the pan with some fat from the sausage or grease well with oil, butter, or ghee to prevent the quiche from sticking.

12. Pour the mixture into the cast iron pan or oven-safe dish.

13. Bake for 40-45 minutes or until a knife poked at the center comes out clean.

14. Serve and enjoy while warm.

Spinach Omelet

Ingredients:

- 2 egg whites
- 1 egg
- 1/2 cup fresh spinach

Instructions:

1. Put together beaten egg and egg whites, whilst forming a "pocket-like" shape.
2. Load the pocket with spinach. Cook until the spinach is wilted. Season with salt and pepper.
3. Serve immediately.

Spinach Berry Lemon Smoothie

Ingredients:

- 2 cups fresh spinach leaves, rinsed and roughly chopped
- 7–8 frozen strawberries
- 1 tbsp. chia seeds
- 1 tbsp. lemon juice
- 1 frozen banana, sliced
- 2–3 cups coconut water, chilled

Instructions:

1. Put the spinach leaves into the blender.
2. Add the banana, strawberries, lemon juice, chia seeds, and coconut water.
3. Blend well.
4. Serve and enjoy!

Avocado, Cucumber, and Tomato Salad

Ingredients:

- 1/4 cup extra-virgin olive oil
- 1 pc. lemon, juiced
- 1/4 tsp. cumin, ground
- salt, to taste
- freshly ground black pepper, to taste
- 3 medium avocados, cubed
- 1-pint cherry tomatoes, halved
- 1 small cucumber, sliced into half-moons
- 1/3 cup corn
- 2 tbsp. cilantro, chopped

Instructions:

1. Combine avocados, cilantro, corn, cucumber, jalapeño, and tomatoes in a large bowl.
2. In a separate small container, whisk together lemon juice, cumin, and oil to make the salad dressing.
3. Season the dressing with salt and pepper.
4. Toss the salad gently while adding the dressing.
5. Serve immediately.

Fruit Salad with Zesty Vinaigrette

Ingredients:

- 3 mangoes, medium-sized, peeled and sliced thinly
- 3 ripe avocados, medium-sized, peeled and thinly sliced
- 1 cup blackberries, fresh
- 1 cup raspberries, fresh
- 1/4 cup mint, fresh and minced
- 1/4 cup almonds, toasted and sliced

For the dressing:

- 1 tsp. grated tangerine or orange peel
- 1/2 cup olive oil
- 1/2 tsp. salt
- 1/4 cup tangerine or orange juice
- 1/4 tsp. freshly ground pepper
- 2 tbsp. balsamic vinegar

Instructions:

1. Combine all the fruits on a serving plate.
2. Sprinkle the salad with mint and almonds.
3. Whisk together all the dressing ingredients in a smaller bow.
4. Drizzle the dressing over the salad.
5. Consume after serving.

Chicken Salad

Ingredients:

- 1 small can of premium chunk chicken breast packed in water
- 1 stalk celery, large, finely chopped
- 1/4 cup reduced-fat mayonnaise
- 4 romaine leaves or red leaf lettuce, washed and trimmed
- 8 pcs. cherry tomatoes or 1 ripe tomato, quartered
- 1 cucumber, small and sliced thinly

Instructions:

1. Drain canned chicken and transfer to a bowl.
2. Put in celery and mayonnaise.
3. Mix lightly. Don't crush the chicken.
4. In a separate shallow bowl, place the lettuce neatly.
5. Add the chicken salad in the middle
6. Add tomatoes and cucumber slices to the plate.
7. Refrigerate before serving, cover with plastic wrap.

Chicken Broth

Ingredients:

- 1 chicken carcass from a leftover roast chicken or bones
- 2 cloves of garlic
- water
- Optional: carrot or parsnip tops, leftover vegetable peelings, and herbs

Instructions:

1. Cover chicken bones with water, whether cooking in a large stockpot, a pressure cooker, or a slow cooker.
2. For the slow cooker, cook on high for 4 hours.
3. For the pressure cooker, set it to cook for an hour.
4. For the stockpot, set it on a low simmer for 3 to 4 hours.
5. Once the time is up, strain the liquid from the broth through a sieve into a large bowl or container.
6. Discard the bones and garlic.
7. Keep the liquid, and pour it into a container.

Roasted Chicken Thighs

Ingredients:

- 12 garlic cloves, unpeeled
- 1 tbsp. avocado oil
- 1 pinch Himalayan pink salt
- 4 chicken thighs with skin
- 1 tsp. Primal Palate super gyro seasoning

Instructions:

1. Pour avocado oil over a medium-sized oven-safe pot.
2. Add the garlic cloves. Sauté over medium heat for 2 to 3 minutes or until the skins begin to brown.
3. Place the chicken in a large skillet over medium-high heat. Sear for about 2 to 3 minutes for each side, starting with the skin side.
4. Combine the chicken with the garlic. Season generously with salt and Primal Palate Super Gyro seasoning.
5. Place the chicken in an oven preheated to 350°F.
6. Bake for one hour while covered.
7. Serve and enjoy.

Sesame Chicken

Ingredients:

Coating & Chicken:

- 1 egg
- 1 lb. chicken thighs, cut into bite-sized pieces
- 1 tbsp. arrowroot powder
- 1 tbsp. toasted sesame seed oil
- salt
- pepper

Sesame Sauce:

- 1 tbsp. toasted sesame seed oil
- 1 tbsp. vinegar
- 2 tbsp. soy sauce
- ginger, cubed into 1 cm
- 2 tbsp. Sukrin Gold
- 2 tbsp. sesame seeds
- 1/4 tsp. xanthan gum
- 1 clove garlic

Instructions:

1. Combine and whisk well egg and arrowroot powder.
2. Place chicken thigh pieces in.
3. In a large frying pan, heat up sesame seed oil.
4. Cook the chicken pieces. Make sure there are gaps between the meat.

5. In a bowl, combine and whisk all the ingredients for the sauce.
6. After cooking all the chicken pieces, pour in the sesame sauce to the pan. Stir and cook for about 5 more minutes, or until the sauce thickens.
7. Transfer chicken on top of cooked broccoli.
8. Upon serving, sprinkle with green onion and sesame seeds.

Grilled Flank Steak

Ingredients:

- 3 lbs. flank steak, cut into bite-sized pieces
- 1 cup coconut oil or olive oil
- 1 lemon, juice only
- 1/2 cup apple cider vinegar
- 2/3 cup coconut aminos
- 2 tbsp. mustard
- 6 cloves of garlic, crushed
- 1 tbsp. fresh ginger, grated
- 1 tbsp. paprika
- 1 tbsp. dried onion, chopped; substitute with onion powder
- 1 tbsp. salt
- 2 tsp. dried thyme
- 1 tsp. chili powder

Instructions:

1. Using all the ingredients except for the steak, create the marinade by mixing everything.
2. Use olive oil if marinating overnight. Use melted coconut oil if marinating for an hour only at room temperature.

3. Place each piece of steak into a Ziploc bag and divide the marinade equally between the bags. Seal the bags and marinate for an hour or overnight.
4. Grill and serve while hot.

Shrimp Avocado Salad

Ingredients:

Salad:

- 1/2 lb. large shrimp, peeled
- 2 sweet corn ears, removed from the cob
- 4 cups Romaine lettuce, chopped
- 3 strips of bacon, diced
- 1 avocado, peeled, pitted and diced
- Optional: 1/3 cup Fontina cheese, grated

Buttermilk pesto dressing:

- 1/2 cup buttermilk
- 1/4 cup pesto, homemade or store-bought
- 1/2 cup mayo or Greek yogurt
- 1 tbsp. lemon juice
- 1 small shallot, minced
- salt
- pepper

Instructions:

1. Over high heat, place a skillet.
2. Put in the corn kernels when the skillet heats up.
3. Allow to dry roast while stirring occasionally. Cook until the edges start to caramelize and turn brown, or for about 6-8 minutes.
4. Place the roasted corn on a plate and set aside.

5. Lower the heat to medium-high. Fry the bacon using the same skillet, for about 6 minutes, until crispy.
6. Transfer the bacon to a plate.
7. Saute the shrimp in the same skillet until they are cooked.
8. In a bowl, toss the lettuce, corn, avocado, bacon, and shrimp.
9. Whisk all the ingredients together until blended.
10. Season with salt and pepper.

Baked Wild Salmon

Ingredients:

- 1.5 lbs. wild salmon
- 2 tbsp. olive oil
- 3 cloves garlic, minced
- 1 tsp. dried oregano
- sea salt
- pepper
- 1 bunch fresh asparagus
- 1/2 cup cucumber
- 1/2 cup tomato, diced
- 1/2 cup feta cheese
- 1/2 cup olives
- 1 whole lemon

Instructions:

1. Preheat the oven to 400°F.
2. Line a baking sheet with parchment paper and set aside.
3. Using a small glass bowl, mix oil, oregano, salt, garlic, and pepper. Pour seasoning mix over the salmon and coat the entire fish.
4. Layer the salmon on the baking sheet.
5. Place trimmed asparagus on the sheet pan next to the salmon.

6. Squeeze fresh lemon juice and place the remaining lemon slices on the sheet pan. Bake for 20 minutes.
7. When the salmon is done, serve with a scoop of olive and feta salad over the salmon or on the side and enjoy.

Smoked Salmon and Baked Eggs in Avocado

Ingredients:

- 4 oz. smoked salmon
- 8 eggs
- 4 avocados, halved and deseeded
- fresh dill
- red chili flakes
- salt
- black pepper

Instructions:

1. Preheat the oven to 425°F.
2. In preparing the avocado, make sure that the hole where the seed was can fit an egg. Carve it out more if needed.
3. Place the avocados on a baking sheet.
4. Put smoked salmon strips on each hollow.
5. Crack open an egg in a small bowl. Spoon out the yolk and the white and transfer to the avocado. Carefully eyeball how much egg the avocado can hold.
6. Sprinkle the avocado with salt and pepper.
7. Bake in the oven for about 15-20 minutes.
8. Top with dill and chili flakes upon serving.

Salmon and Asparagus

Ingredients:

- 2 salmon filets
- 14-oz. young potatoes
- 8 asparagus spears, trimmed and halved
- 2 handfuls cherry tomatoes
- 1 handful basil leaves
- 2 tbsp. extra-virgin olive oil
- 1 tbsp. balsamic vinegar

Instructions:

1. Heat oven to 428°F.
2. Arrange potatoes into a baking dish.
3. Drizzle potatoes with extra-virgin olive oil.
4. Roast potatoes until they have turned golden brown.
5. Place asparagus into the baking dish together with the potatoes.
6. Roast in the oven for 15 minutes.
7. Arrange cherry tomatoes and salmon among the vegetables.
8. Drizzle with balsamic vinegar and the remaining olive oil.
9. Roast until the salmon is cooked.
10. Throw in basil leaves before transferring everything to a serving dish.
11. Serve while hot.

Kale Banana Smoothie

Ingredients:

- 16 oz. coconut water, chilled
- 1 pc. banana
- half avocado, peeled and sliced
- 1/2 cup kale
- 1/8 lemon juice
- a pinch of cayenne pepper

Instructions:

1. Blend all the ingredients until smooth.
2. Put it in a glass then serve.

Fruity Berry Spinach Smoothie

Ingredients:

- 1 cup watermelon
- 1 cup almond milk
- 1/2 small banana
- 1 handful of spinach
- 5 frozen strawberries
- 1 tsp. chia seeds
- 1 cup ice

Instructions:

1. Mix spinach, banana, chia seeds, half cup of ice, and half cup of almond milk. Do this to prevent a brown smoothie.
2. Pour into a glass.
3. Blend the rest of the ingredients.
4. Pour both of the mixtures into the same glass.
5. Serve and enjoy!

Muesli-Style Oatmeal

Ingredients:

- 1/2 banana, diced
- 1 cup instant oatmeal
- 1/2 golden apple, peeled and diced
- 1 cup milk
- 2 tbsp. raisins
- 2 tsp. honey or sugar
- A pinch of salt

Instructions:

1. In a bowl, mix oatmeal, raisins, milk, sugar or honey, and salt.
2. Put on a cover and refrigerate.
3. Leave the mixture overnight or for at least 2 hours.
4. Get it out of the fridge after the allotted time then serve it with fruits.
5. Add some milk if the mixture gets too thick.
6. Serve while warm.

Conclusion

Processed food addiction may seem difficult to cure. Yes, it can be challenging but never impossible. By learning to make the right choices and attaining your goal to stay healthy, especially in the long run, you will be able to start over and be free from the addiction.

Thank you for following this beginner's guide to processed food addiction. Remember that it is a process and it might take some time before we see results. Be patient and stay the course—you can do it!

Processed food addiction can be debilitating and scary. However, with the right tools and information, we can overcome it. This beginner's guide provides all of the necessary information to get started on our journey to recovery. Remember to stay patient, take things one step at a time, and reach out for help when needed. You are worth it!

If you enjoyed this guide, please share it with your friends and family. And don't forget to leave a review.

References and Helpful Links

"Ultra-processed" foods make up more than half of all calories in US diet: And contribute 90 percent of all dietary added sugar intake. (n.d.). ScienceDaily. Retrieved November 20, 2022, from https://www.sciencedaily.com/releases/2016/03/160309202154.htm.

10 processed foods to cut down on. (n.d.). BBC Good Food. Retrieved November 20, 2022, from https://www.bbcgoodfood.com/health/processed-foods-avoid.

12 common food additives—Should you avoid them? (2018, April 23). Healthline. https://www.healthline.com/nutrition/common-food-additives.

A narrative review of highly processed food addiction across the lifespan. (n.d.). Retrieved November 20, 2022, from https://www.researchgate.net/publication/346449916_A_narrative_revie w_of_highly_processed_food_addiction_across_the_lifespan.

Eating highly processed foods linked to weight gain. (2019, May 20). National Institutes of Health (NIH). https://www.nih.gov/news-events/nih-research-matters/eating-highly-pro cessed-foods-linked-weight-gain.

Eating processed foods. (2022, February 23). NHS.UK. https://www.nhs.uk/live-well/eat-well/how-to-eat-a-balanced-diet/what-a re-processed-foods/.

Lustig, R. H. (2020). Ultraprocessed food: Addictive, toxic, and ready for regulation. Nutrients, 12(11), 3401. https://doi.org/10.3390/nu12113401.

Opioids and the Brain—How do changes in the brain begin? (2019, April 10). PursueCare. https://www.pursuecare.com/opioids-and-the-brain/.

Processed foods: Health risks and what to avoid. (2020, May 15). https://www.medicalnewstoday.com/articles/318630.

Read •Health, S. this to read later S. to email 5 M. & Wellness. (2019, January 15). Excess sugar consumption: Is it ruining your health? NewYork-Presbyterian. https://healthmatters.nyp.org/how-much-sugar-is-too-much/.

Resource grains. (n.d.). Retrieved November 20, 2022, from https://foodbuyingguide.fns.usda.gov/FoodComponents/ResourceGrains.

Salt appetite is linked to drug addiction, research finds. (n.d.). ScienceDaily. Retrieved November 20, 2022, from https://www.sciencedaily.com/releases/2011/07/110711151451.htm.

Services, D. of H. & H. (n.d.). Food additives. Retrieved November 20, 2022, from http://www.betterhealth.vic.gov.au/health/conditionsandtreatments/food-additives.

Steele, E. M., Baraldi, L. G., Louzada, M. L. da C., Moubarac, J.-C., Mozaffarian, D., & Monteiro, C. A. (2016). Ultra-processed foods and added sugars in the US diet: Evidence from a nationally representative cross-sectional study. BMJ Open, 6(3), e009892. https://doi.org/10.1136/bmjopen-2015-009892.

The worst junk foods for your kids. (2013, January 28). ChildrensMD.
https://childrensmd.org/browse-by-age-group/the-worst-junk-foods-for-y
our-kids/.

Underlying mechanisms of highly processed food addiction. (n.d.).
Psychiatric Times. Retrieved November 20, 2022, from
https://www.psychiatrictimes.com/view/underlying-mechanisms-highly-
processed-food-addiction.

What are endorphins? (n.d.). Verywell Mind. Retrieved November 20,
2022, from
https://www.verywellmind.com/what-are-endorphins-5025072.

Printed in the USA
CPSIA information can be obtained
at www.ICGtesting.com
LVHW021108171023
761168LV00028B/257